YOUR KNOWLEDGE HAS VALUE

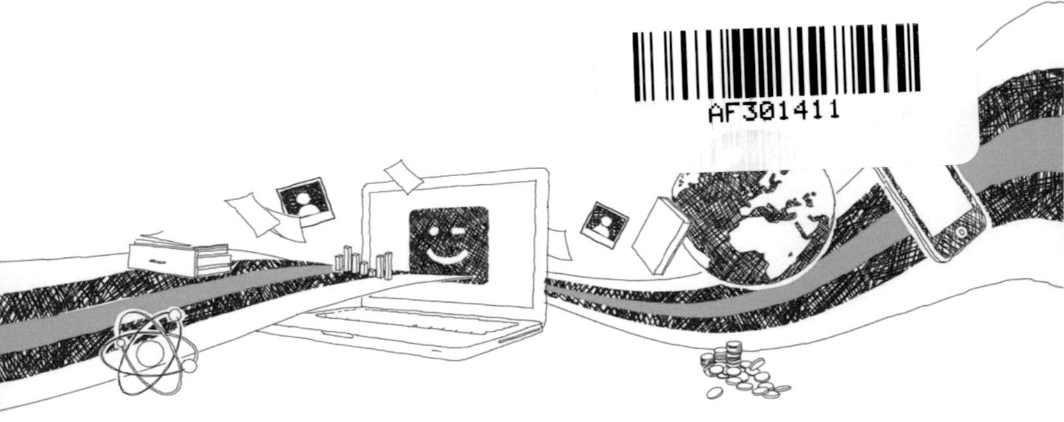

- We will publish your bachelor's and master's thesis, essays and papers

- Your own eBook and book - sold worldwide in all relevant shops

- Earn money with each sale

Upload your text at www.GRIN.com and publish for free

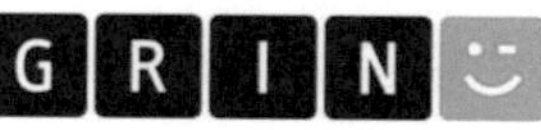

Peter Okeke

The Distribution of ABO Blood Group System

In Porto Novo District Of Cape Verde Islands

GRIN Publishing

Bibliographic information published by the German National Library:

The German National Library lists this publication in the National Bibliography; detailed bibliographic data are available on the Internet at http://dnb.dnb.de .

Imprint:

Copyright © 2009 GRIN Verlag GmbH
Print and binding: Books on Demand GmbH, Norderstedt Germany
ISBN: 978-3-640-79073-9

This book at GRIN:

http://www.grin.com/en/e-book/163580/the-distribution-of-abo-blood-group-system

The Distribution
Of

ABO BLOOD GROUP SYSTEM

In Porto Novo District
Of Cape Verde Islands

By
Okeke Peter Ubah
2009

RESEARCH SEQUENCE:

    Basic structures and nature of ABO blood group system antigens
A and B red cell antigens
Nature of ABO blood group system antibodies
Frequency of occurrence of ABO groups
Importance of ABO blood group system

    Materials
ABO blood grouping method

Aims and Objectives

This work basically has an objective to find the frequency of occurrence of the ABO blood group system in Porto Novo population. It also tells which group of blood is common among the population and which group is rare in the Porto Novo people.

The research work will go a long way to serve in the future for a partial fulfilment of a degree program in health science (Haematology with transfusion science) of the **Atlantic International University (AIU) Honolulu – Hawaii.**

ACKNOWLEDGEMENTS

I am deeply grateful to Dr. Emmanuel Mba chief Laboratory Haematologist working in Ontario Canada who first took me into the medical technology profession.

Secondly, special thanks goes to Dr. José Brito, a general physician working at the central hospital Porto Novo who continued and persistently show interests in laboratory aspect of medicine and some of his valuable advice has been noted.

However, I sincerely thank Mr. Erineu Oliveira Rodrigues of the branch office of the Ministry of Education Porto Novo for his valuable help and computer typing of the various section of this work.

City of Porto Novo, 2009

ABSTRACT

A total of 750 blood samples were collected into the dipotassium – ethylene diaminetetra – acetic acid (EDTA) tubes and BD vacutainer tubes from the population of Porto Novo at random ranging from 2 years to 70 years of age. The ABO blood group systems were tested on the samples by the forward and reverse technique of blood grouping by tube method.

A total of 320 individuals were shown to be blood group O (43%), the blood group A were shown to be 226 individuals (30%), blood group B were 167 people (22%) and blood AB finally were 37 people making up to 5% of the population tested. This work follows almost the same discovery made by other researchers of ABO grouping system and did not show a significant differences among the groups except in that reported on Brazilian Indians in Mato Grosso which registered 100% blood group O among Indians of Mato Grosso by Bier at al(1982).

The work serves as a fundamental screening on the distribution of ABO blood group system in Porto Novo and did not indicate whether there exists a difference of ABO blood group system distribution among other islands of Cape Verde and also a reference point for those engaged in clinical blood use like the red cross organisation and paramedical units who at times give blood on emergency basis.

INTRODUCTION TO ABO BLOOD GROUP SYSTEM

The importance of the ABO blood group systems in blood transfusion lies in the frequency of their antibodies. The ABO system was the first to be recognised and remains the most important.

The vast majority of transfusion accidents that cause serious patient injury are due to an error in identifying patient samples or donor units that result in the transfusion of an ABO incompatible blood or its product. A significant number of Transfusion accidents occur however, due to ABO typing errors in the transfusion Laboratory which has resulted in many deaths.

The ABO typing test is therefore the most critical procedure encountered and performed in any given blood bank laboratory.

BASIC STRUCTURES AND NATURE OF ABO BLOOD GROUP SYSTEM ANTIGENS

The presence or absence of two antigens (A and B) defines the four blood types of the ABO blood group system. The ABO blood groups are determined genetically by the inheritance of a gene or genes that code for the production of transferase enzymes.

These enzymes are called "glycosyltransferases" which add specific hexoses (6 carbon sugars) to oligosaccharide chains present on the RBC membrane. In a series of enzymatic reactions, the ABH antigens are formed.

The first of these enzyme reactions is the addition of fucose to oligosaccharide chains on the red cell membrane by the action of Fucosyltransferase produced by the H gene. This creates the H-antigen structure that is the substrate for further transferase activity associated with the A and B genes.

The two other genetically controlled enzymes, the group A transferase (N – acetylgalactosaminyl transferase) and the group B transferase (D – galactosyltransferase) control the addition of the terminal sugars N-acetylgalactosamine and D – galactose respectively to the oligosaccharide chain that has acquired H – antigen specificity.

However, a persons ABO blood group depends on the A, B, or O gene located on chromosome 9, inherited from each parent as follows:

Genes inherited (genotype)	Blood group (Phenotype)
A and A A and O	Group A
B and B B and O	Group B
A and B	Group AB
O and O	Group O

A and B genes are dominant. The recessive O gene is expressed only when A and B dominant gene are absent. A person who is group O must be of the genotype OO.

A AND B RED CELL ANTIGENS

A person who inherits A gene (AA and AO) belongs to group A and expresses A antigen on their red cells.

A person who inherits B gene (BB and BO) belongs to group B and express B antigen on their red cells.

A person who inherits A and B genes belongs to group AB and express both A and B antigens on their red cells.

A person who inherits O genes belongs to group O and does not express any antigens (A or B) on their red cells.

NATURE OF ABO BLOOD GROUP SYSTEM ANTIBODIES

ABO blood group system antibodies are significantly different from those directed at other blood group system antigens because they are potent, naturally occurring antibodies found universally in immunocompetent persons.

Current thinking indicates that the A and B antigen structure on red blood cell membrane is similar to bacterial antigen structures found in the environment, these bacterial antigens stimulate production of the naturally occurring antibodies of the ABO blood group system.

However, in addition to naturally environmental stimulation, immune antibodies of the ABO system may be produced after exposure to foreign red blood cells.

Thus, individuals lacking A antigen produce Anti-A antibodies and those lacking B antigen produce Anti-B antibodies. Group O individuals lack both A and B antigen and thus produce anti-A and anti-B antibodies, were as group AB persons have both A and B antigens and produce no ABO antibodies. Group AB otherwise could be regarded as an inert serum, having no A+B antibodies.

FREQUENCY OF OCCURRENCE OF ABO GROUPS

Before talking on the frequency of blood systems of the ABO, it is a common practice in the world today to test for compatibility before blood or its product is given. However some authorities still think that group O blood is simply a universal donor and at such group O blood could be given to A, B or AB recipients freely without hindrance at all. In today's context, there are some group O persons who are termed "DANGEROUS UNIVERSAL DONORS".

However, group O donors have anti-A and anti-B in their plasma which theoretically would agglutinate the recipients A or B cells. Normally, if these are naturally occurring antibodies, they will be diluted out and neutralized by the plasma of the adult recipients.

If they are immune antibodies, this neutralization and dilution effect could be insufficient and can lead to marked destruction of the A or B red cells of the person receiving it and can cause severe transfusion reactions and sometimes may lead to death of the recipients. Therefore it has become imperative for the users of blood transfusion to seek for knowledge for alternative transfusion currently going on in the world today, knowing fully well that the best transfusion is the transfusion never given.

The incidence of ABO blood groups varies very markedly in different parts of the world.

Dr. Herzfeld et al (1919) reported early studies on the anthropology of the ABO system and stated that the distribution geographically and racially of these blood group ABO, offer a special interests to researchers in the direct application to anthropology and genetics.

Dobson and IKin (1946) observed that in Northern England blood group O is 47% of population, the blood group AB is only 3% of the population of Northern England. Dobson and IKin also reported that Southern England showed 43% of blood group O and group AB is 0.64% to 2.62% of the population. It is striking therefore to note that as small as the United Kingdom is, there exists a profound difference in distribution of ABO systems.

That blood group AB dominate in parts of Asia. According to Dr. Lozza, blood group O is very high among primitive Americans (Indians and esquimos), Islander and Philippines.

Dr Lozza observed that Europeans generally have predominate blood group A against blood group O and blood group AB among Europeans do not and cannot pass 5% of European population.

Soares et al (1985) reported that blood group B has major occurrence between the people of Asian with China having 27% of blood group B while Hindus showed 37%.

The interesting work of Bier, Mota, Vaz and Dias da Silva (1982) on Brazilian population is shown below:

Blood Group	Brazilian whites%	Brazilian blacks%	Brazilian Indians%
O	45	49	100
A	41	25	-
B	10	22	-
AB	4	4	-

The work of Bier, Mota, Vaz and Dias da Silva (1982) was in accord with that of offensooser et al (1950) on Brazilian primitive Indians having blood group O 100% of their population. It is worthy to note that both Brazilian blacks and whites showed 4% of blood group AB while whites having higher percentage of 41% blood group A against blacks with only 25%.

Dr Vengelen (1996) reported that group O blood group was 79% in the Native Americans. He also expressed that the American Whites have group O to be 45% compared to the United States blacks with 49% blood group O.
Dr Vengelen (1996) once again reported that both whites and blacks living in the United States of America have blood group AB to be 4%.

Monica Cheesbrough (2000) reported that the blacks in African continent showed blood group O 49% and blood group A among black Africans was 26%, the report also showed blood group B 21% and blood group AB of blacks of American continent was 4% of the population tested.

Monica Cheesbrough (2000) also stated that among Nepalese, blood group A was 33% where as blood group B was 27% of the population tested in Nepal. The people of origin Caucasian has the same distribution of blood group AB equal to African blacks of the African continent both 4% respectively.

Monica (2000) still on Nepalese did mention that 12% of the population of Nepalese tested was blood group AB. All this indicates that different races present a predominance of ABO blood groups relative to others.

IMPORTANCE OF ABO BLOOD GROUP SYSTEM

ABO blood group system is widely applicable in anthropology, genetics and transfusion medicine. It is also important in a transfusion of same blood products and constitutes a case study of materno-fetal incompatibility in obstetrics. ABO blood group system is the basics of fundamental medico – legal medicine where exists the problem of percentage and or paternity dispute. The determination of blood group antigens of ABO can do no more than to exclude one of the two disputing parents, and in most cases could be 15 to 25% probability.

However, the man (suspecting father) is always in dispute and the main principles governing exclusion from paternity is that firstly the man (suspecting father) is excluded if both he and the mother of the child lack an antigen which is present in the child. The man once again is excluded if the antigens which the man (suspecting father) must pass on to the child is absent.

Although, ABO blood group system determination alone is not sufficient for paternity dispute without considering other advanced procedures such as DNA determination but it could serve as a starting point to all other important techniques relating to this material.

MATERIALS AND METHOD

MATERIALS

1. 750 blood samples were collected at random starting from 2 years old person to about 70 years old from both sexes. Clotted and EDTA samples.
2. Small test tubes (65 x 9.5 mm).
3. Antisera: Anti – A, Anti – B and Anti – A+B.
4. 2 to 5% cells suspensions; A – cells, B – cells, O – cells, all freshly pooled.
5. Test tube racks.
6. Pasteur pipettes.
7. Times with alarm system.
8. Room thermometer.
9. 9g/L Nacl (saline)
10. Tubes of Dipotassium ethylenediamine tetra acetic acid (EDTA)

ABO BLOOD GROUPING METHOD

The tube method is the method of choice and is particularly suitable when grouping large numbers of samples. For example in this study a total of 750 blood samples were tested.

The patient's red cells and serum are both grouped and the two results compared.

Anti-A, Anti-B and Anti A+ B (group – O) sera are used for the cell grouping tests. Pooled A, B and O – cells are used for the serum grouping tests.

The anti-A+B serum acts as an additional check on blood samples which are agglutinated by anti-A or anti-B and it should also detect the rare types of A cells which may not be agglutinated by the anti-A found in group-B people.

The room temperature of 18 to 25ºc was maintained throughout the test. The antiserum used in the study was avid and or potent so as to cause rapid, intense and clear cut observable reaction.

TECHNIQUE

Add by means of a Pasteur Pipette, I drop of each grouping serum to 3 tubes labelled Anti-A, Anti-B and Anti – A+B respectively.

This was followed by I drop of 2 to 5% cell suspension in saline (9 glL Nacl) of the test cells.

Additionally I volume of the person's serum was added to 4 tubes labelled A-cells, B – cells, O – cells and auto agglutination control respectively. Then I volume of 2 to 5% cell suspensions of the control A, B and O cells appropriate tubes.

Mix the suspensions by tapping the tubes and leave them undisturbed in the laboratory for 1 ½ to 2 hrs results are based on agglutination and or haemolysis.

Presence of agglutination and or haemolysis is considered as positive and its absence as negative respectively. Apparently all negative results were checked with the aid of low power microscope.

Each grouping test or series of tests were controlled by parallel tests set up exactly as described above, using cells of known blood group in place of the test cells.

RESULTS

The results of ABO group system performed on a total of 750 individuals at random between the ages of 2 to 70 years are shown below:

Table 1.1

The ABO blood group system frequencies (in percent) of Porto Novo population.

Blood group	Frequency of occurrence in percent
O	43
A	30
B	22
AB	5

Table 1.2

Blood group histogram showing frequency distribution in percent

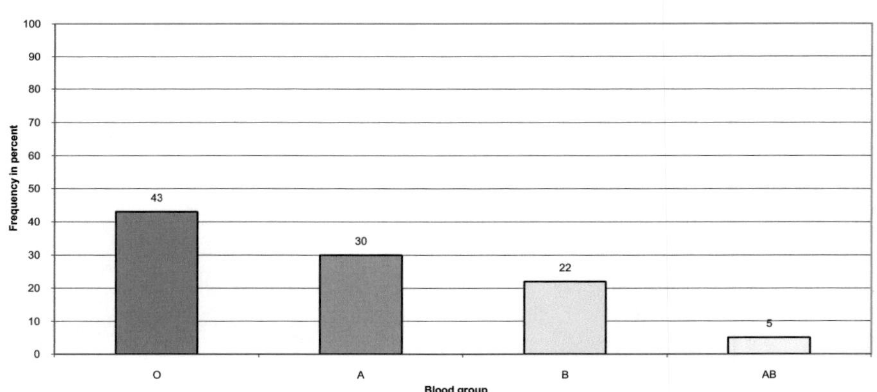

DISCUSSION

The results of the ABO blood group system analyzed on a total of 750 individuals expressed blood group O as the group with major occurrences with 320 people expressing blood group O, a percentage of 43% of the total number tested. The blood group A was 226 persons also accounting for 30%. The blood group B was 167 persons making a 22 % and blood group AB with 37 persons amounting to 5% of the population tested.

However, blood group dominant in the city of Porto Novo and its affiliated towns and villages has shown clearly to be blood group O while blood group AB is the most rare blood group system in Porto Novo district.

The work of Vengelen et al (1996) on American population of the United States reported blood group O with 49% among the United States Negroes and 79% among Native Americans. Vengelen at al (1996) was not totally in contrast with Porto Novo ABO distribution, but showed a little difference between 43% of blood group O in Porto Novo and that of 49% among USA Negroes and contrasted with that of Native Americans with 79%.

Further more in line with Porto Novo blood group distribution was the work of Monica (2000) which expressed 49% of blood group O among African Negroes resident in Africa and group AB of African Negroes was 4%.we could see clearly that the grouping system in Porto Novo follows almost the same pattern.

However, the Porto Novo distribution was directly in agreement in part with the report of Bier Mota and Dias da Silva et al (1982) on Brazilian Negroes living in Brazil and they reported blood group B up to 22% of the population tested in Brazil. We might recall that blood group B distribution in Porto Novo was 22% recorded in this work, but the work of Bier et al differs greatly on blood group O (100%) reported on Brazilian Indians of Mato Grosso, while that of Porto Novo population according to this research was 43%. The Porto Novo ABO distribution experience also agreed once again in part to that of southern England of Great Britain reported by Dobson and IKin (1946) in which blood group O distribution of southern England was 43% equal to the blood group O seen among Porto Novo residence also 43%. The experience of Dobson and IKin (1946) differs a little with that of Porto Novo in blood group B (8%) distribution and group AB 2.62% of the southern England people compared to Porto Novo blood group B (22%) and group AB (5%).

There could also be environmental factors in effect to the formation of blood group antigens and different races present different ABO blood group distribution and inheritance.

However, whether there exists ABO distribution differences between Porto Novo and Praia or similarities between city of Porto Portugal and city of Porto Novo Cape Verde is still unclear.

It is worthy to observe the ABO blood group distribution similarities between Porto Novo and some parts of the world.

Finally, the ABO blood group system of Porto Novo is now a scientific reality in terms of its frequency distribution among the population residing in the city of Porto Novo and its environs and we could not fail to say that it almost follows the same pattern as observed in most parts of the world.

Conclusion

In conclusion, it is clear to note that the blood group dominant in Porto novo province is blood group O with 43%, secondly with blood group A 30%, thirdly blood group B with 22% and then blood group AB with 5% respectively. The grouping follows the same distribution made in other areas with little differences and some areas with equal distribution. The grouping of ABO continued to be the most relevant test done in Hospital transfusion practice and as such is necessary to establish it´s distribution in a given population which will go a long way to help in it´s application by the Red Cross and other paramedical services constantly engaged with emergency situation involving the clinical use of blood.

REFERENCES

1. Allen F. H.:
    Importance of the blood groups in laboratory and clinical medicine. New England. I. Medicine 247; 379, 1952.

2. Baker, Silverton and Pallister:
    Introduction to Medical Laboratory Technology 7th edn. P. 399, 1998

3. Batfaglia. A;
    Grupos Sanguineous en la Poblácion de Buenos Aires. Rev. Soc. Arg. Hemat & Hemot .I. 169; 1949.

4. Bhende. Y. M. et al;
    A new blood character related to the ABO system. Lancet, 1: 903, 1952.

5. Bier, O. G. et al:
    Imunologia Básica e Aplicada, 3rd ed. Rio de Janeiro, Editora Guanabara Koagan S. A. 1982.

6. Chalmers J. N. M. et al:
    Basic blood groups, Nature 162: 27, 1948.

7. Dobson. A. And IKin E. W;
    The ABO blood group in the United Kingdom frequencies based on a very large sample J. Path. Bact. 58, 221; 1946.

8. Dunsford and Bowley:
    Techniques in blood grouping 2nd edn voll. II, p. 270 (b) p. 354. Oliver and Boyd Edinburgh.

9. Ervin D. M. et al:
    Dangerous Universal Donors Blood 5: 553, 1950

10. Giblett. E. R.:
    A critique of the theoretical hazard of Inter vs. Intraracial Transfusion, 1. 233, 1961

11. Herzfeld. L.: Les Groups Sanguins
    Paris, Masson & Cie
    Editeurs, 1938.

12. Issitt. P. D.:
    Applied Blood Group Serology, Miami, Montgomery Scientific Publications, 1985.

13. Lynch. M. J. et al:
    Medical Laboratory Technology and Clinical Pathology.

Philadelphia, London and Toronto W. B. Saunders, Co. 1969.

14. Monica Cheesbrough (2002):
District Laboratory Practice in Tropical Countries Vol. II, Blood Transfusion Tests, P. 363.

15. Mollison P. L. et al:
Blood transfusion in Clinical Medicine. 10th ed. Oxford Blackwell Scientific Pub. 1997.

16.   Offensooser et al:
Tipos Sanguineos de Indios do Mato Grosso,
O Hospital 37:73, 1950

17. Race R. R. et al:
Blood groups in man 6th edn. Blackwell scientific Pub. Oxford and Edinburg.

18. Rudmann. S. V. et al:
Textbook of Blood Banking and Transfusion Medicine, Philadelphia W. B. Saunders 1995.

19. Soares et al;
Métodos de Laboratório aplicadas à Clinica, Técnica e Interpretação 1985, p. 359.

20. Vengelen Tyler et al:
Technical Manual, 12th edn, Bethesda, M. D. American Association of Blood Banks. 1996 p. 230.